SEX Guide For Men

Orgasm Manual - Shoot Her To The Moon And Back

By: More Sex More Fun Book Club

© **Copyright 2017 - All rights reserved.**
In no way is it legal to reproduce, duplicate, or transmit any part of this document in either electronic means or in printed format. Recording of this publication is strictly prohibited and any storage of this document is not allowed unless with written permission from the publisher. All rights reserved.

The information provided herein is stated to be truthful and consistent, in that any liability, in terms of inattention or otherwise, by any usage or abuse of any policies, processes, or directions contained within is the solitary and utter responsibility of the recipient reader. Under no circumstances will any legal responsibility or blame be held against the publisher for any reparation, damages, or monetary loss due to the information herein, either directly or indirectly.
Respective authors own all copyrights not held by the publisher.

Legal Notice:
This book is copyright protected. This is only for personal use. You cannot amend, distribute, sell, use, quote or paraphrase any part or the content within this book without the consent of the author or copyright owner. Legal action will be pursued if this is breached.

Disclaimer Notice:
Please note the information contained within this document is for educational and entertainment purposes only. Every attempt has been made to provide accurate, up to date and reliable complete information. No warranties of any kind are expressed or implied. Readers acknowledge that the author is not engaging in the rendering of legal, financial, medical or professional advice.

By reading this document, the reader agrees that under no circumstances are we responsible for any losses, direct or indirect, which are incurred as a result of the use of information contained within this document, including, but not limited to, —errors, omissions, or inaccuracies.

Table of Contents

Introduction	1
Chapter 1: The History Of The Female Orgasm	3
Chapter 2: The Ins And Outs Of The Female Orgasm	6
Chapter 3: Types Of Female Orgasms	14
Chapter 4: Make Her Come	18
Chapter 5: Positions That Will Work For Her Every Time	22
Chapter 6: Additional Tips To Help Both Of You Out	31
Chapter 7: Myths About Female Orgasms	36
Chapter 8: Solo Play	40
Chapter 9: Getting the Best Orgasm of Your Life	49
Conclusion	51

Introduction

Ah, the orgasm! That sexual ideal and destination which pretty much all men seem to reach, but which seems to remain elusive for plenty of women. It has, in turn, frustrated, excited and confounded but always fascinated the human mind. It has thrown up controversies, shown shocking new facts and made us look at female sexuality very differently over the ages.

But academic interest isn't what is going to help us achieve that much-longed for state of ecstacy. More importantly, it isn't going to get our partner there. So, do you find yourself wondering whether your lover is satisfied in bed? Perhaps you feel that you aren't doing enough to make your sexual life appealing to her. Perhaps you feel that you could do more. Have you wondered whether she faked her orgasm the last time you had sex?

Questions like these about an activity as intimate and closely related to our self-esteem as sex can cause several confidence-killing thoughts. That is where this book comes in. We will examine the female orgasm and all its types in great detail. But this isn't just a technical study. Oh no, that wouldn't help our cause at all. This book is about how to ensure that you and your partner enjoy making love and both of you get maximum pleasure from the act.

We will look at different techniques, old and new. We will examine mental states and how they affect a woman's ability to orgasm. We will learn the effects of communication and lack thereof in terms of a satisfying sexual encounter or a sex life. Most of all, we will look at how you and your partner can have a happier, healthier and more rewarding sexual life.

You don't have to wait to finish the book to start using the advice I give you here. You can start incorporating the changes I recommend as soon as you read them. The point here is to give you a guide that helps you understand your partner's sexual wants, use that understanding to improve your sex life and feel much more satisfied by it than you may feel at the moment.

Thank you for buying this book. I hope you have a pleasant time reading (and following) it.

Chapter 1: The History Of The Female Orgasm

Before we get to how you can pleasure your partner into sexual oblivion, you must understand the way the female orgasm has been perceived throughout the centuries. You may not be aware of it, but the way the big O has been seen with regards to women may have colored your thinking too. While it is a history of repression, it is not solely so. The female orgasm has also gone through periods where great interest was shown. However, only now is it even remotely close to being understood.

Contrary to popular belief, during the medieval times, the female orgasm was considered absolutely necessary to procreation. Medieval scientists believed that a woman needed to orgasm in order to be able to have a child. From the 13th century onwards, the scientific theory held that for the sexual act to be fruitful, a woman must climax during the act. The notion was based on the belief that a woman's sexual organs were exactly like a man's, but they were inverted. This meant that women ejaculated just as men did during sex, the only difference being that they ejaculated inwards.

In the 1800s, sexual tension in women was diagnosed as hysteria. It was also known as wandering womb. The condition was thought to be specific to women and hence was also often called female hysteria. It was believed that the condition would drive a woman completely insane unless it was treated. The mode of treatment? Clitoral stimulation. Women were supposed to masturbate in the privacy of their homes. Those women who were unable to climax received genital massages from physicians. Eventually, these physicians went on to invent the vibrator to make their job easier.

The 1940s brought with them Alfred Kinsey's explosive surveys about people's sexual behavior. Suddenly, the female orgasm wasn't a mysterious and perhaps even mythical phenomenon at all. The Kinsey Report showed that 40 percent of the women who were surveyed masturbated and had achieved their first orgasm that way. Other phenomena such as 'wet dreams,' multiple orgasms and the age at which women may lose the ability to orgasm were also discussed in the Report. While certain aspects of the Report have been debunked, it cannot be denied that the Kinsey Report was instrumental in busting a lot of sexual myths, especially as they related to women.

In the 1960s, now that the female orgasm was an established fact, plenty of studies and theories abounded about the necessity of the female orgasm. Various scientists theorized about why women orgasmed. Desmond Morris, in his book, *The Naked Ape*, theorized that the reason the female orgasm developed was so that women could select good mates and fathers based on qualities other than aggression and size, such as intelligence, care, imagination and patience. He also erroneously suggested that the female orgasm was meant to make the woman feel exhausted at the end of sex and keep her horizontal so that the sperm wouldn't leak out.

Other scientists believed that monogamy was not the goal or the reason for the female orgasm – in fact, it was quite the opposite. According to them, it was a way for women to bond with multiple sexual partners. Some others have speculated that the muscular contractions in the vagina during orgasm help conception by sucking up sperm. Others point out that if a woman achieves orgasm during sex, it is more likely that she will indulge in sex again, thus increasing the chances of conception.

Today, while the purpose of the female orgasm is still not clear, its benefits are definitely out there. It has been proved that orgasms in women improve the mood (naturally!), regulate the menstrual cycle, boost the immune system and the white blood cell levels, improve the functioning of the brain and work as great pain relievers.

So read on and find out how you can ensure that your partner enjoys all these benefits while both of you enjoy a stimulating sex life.

Chapter 2: The Ins And Outs Of The Female Orgasm

So, now that we're beginning, the first thing to know is what the female orgasm is all about. The NHS describes the female orgasm as "an intense, pleasurable release of sexual tension. It is accompanied by contractions of the genital muscles. A woman may be able to experience more than one orgasm shortly after the first if she continues to be stimulated."

So far so good. That sounds simple enough, doesn't it? But as you can tell from the previous chapter the female orgasm has been covered in so much myth and has been the subject of so much repression and misinformation that, today, 25% of women aren't even sure that they have achieved climax – either during sex or while masturbating. Quite a few women are sure that they cannot orgasm and a significant number state that they can only experience orgasm during masturbation and not during sexual intercourse.

All these statistics can be pretty daunting for their sexual partners. Therefore, the first thing to do is arm yourself with information. The first step to ensuring that your partner achieves the same satisfaction that you do during sex is to understand all the factors that govern the female orgasm. This is because unlike a man who is able to achieve orgasm only through physical stimulation, a woman's orgasm is affected by a combination of physical and mental factors. Let us take a look at what some of these factors are.

1. **Physiological Factors**

   There are various physiological factors that can contribute to a woman's failure to climax. If you want to ensure that your partner achieves an orgasm during sex, you must be aware of what these factors are.

   a) Age

   Several studies conducted over the past few decades have found that the incidence of anorgasmia or the inability to orgasm is more prevalent among older women. While the reasons for this aren't well known, it is speculated that this happens because of the hormonal changes that happen with age such as a decrease in the level of estrogen and progesterone because of menopause. It is believed that the changes in the hormonal levels affect a woman's ability to achieve orgasm.

   Certain psychological factors may also affect a woman's ability to climax in a sexual encounter as she ages. We will look at these factors in detail a little later.

   b) Testosterone

   Studies conducted on women and their hormonal levels have linked low levels of testosterone to a decreased ability to be aroused sexually and achieve orgasm. Couple this with the fact that about 70 million women around the world take the oral contraceptive pill which also reduces the testosterone levels in the female body, and it is not surprising that many doctors advise their female patients of the unofficial side effect of the pill – namely, a reduced sex drive and even an inability to achieve orgasm.

c) Estrogen

As mentioned earlier, menopause causes the levels of estrogen in the blood to go down. These lowered levels of the hormone have been linked to changes in sensations in the genitals and the blood flow to and from the genital area. In addition, decreased levels of estrogen also affect lubrication in the vagina and a woman's moods – both of which can explain a loss of interest in sex and an inability to achieve orgasm in menopausal and post-menopausal women.

d) Medical Conditions

Medical conditions can also affect a woman's ability to climax during sex. These conditions can cause more difficulty in achieving an orgasm, reduced frequency of orgasms and a change in how orgasms feel. These conditions include but are not limited to rectal disease, cancer, spinal cord injury, depression, anxiety and other such psychological disorders. Even hysterectomies have been known to adversely affect women's ability to orgasm.

e) Medications

Just as the medical conditions listed above can adversely affect a woman's ability to orgasm during intercourse, so too can the medicines required to treat those conditions. For example, women taking mood altering medicines such as anti-depressants used to treat depression, often complain about an inability to climax during sex or even a decreased sex drive. As mentioned above, the oral contraceptive pill has also been linked to a decreased ability to orgasm in women. There are, however, scientists who postulate that the pill actually benefits a woman's sex drive and her ability to climax. So far, both sides have produced inconclusive evidence to support their theories.

f) Physical stimulation

Yup, this one is true lads. Studies have shown that women are much more likely to achieve climax when there is an adequate amount of foreplay involved. Exactly how much foreplay and for how long is different from woman to woman. We will discuss sexual techniques and positions that will maximize her pleasure, later on in the book.

In addition to foreplay, a whopping 95% of women have reported that they were much more likely to orgasm if clitoral stimulation rather than vaginal stimulation was utilized (only 26% in favor of vaginal stimulation).

2. Psychological factors

Apart from the physiological factors listed above, there are a number of psychological factors that can also affect women's ability to orgasm. These factors can arise from upbringing, social taboos, cultural conditioning, parental upbringing, sexual trauma and various other factors. Let's take a look at some of the prominent factors below.

a) Body Issues

It is a fact that most women are unhappy with their bodies in some way or the other. This unhappiness and self-consciousness can intrude during sex and interrupt the build up to a climax. Thoughts can range from disparaging thoughts about one's body (I'm so fat, my breasts are too large/small, I'm too thin) to feelings of shame associated with the genital region (My vagina is too large/too small, I'm not clean so avoid oral sex, I'm too dry). Negative attitudes towards bodily functions that have been ingrained during toilet training tend to persist throughout one's life. This means that a lot of women see their bodies and specifically their genitals as 'dirty'. As such, they feel much more self-conscious during sex and are unable to enjoy the act enough to climax.

b) Negative Attitudes Towards Sex

Growing up, many women acquire distorted views of sex. They get these views from society and from their families. Sex is viewed as bad or immoral. Attitudes towards nudity, sex play and even masturbation are severely negative and shameful and don't just affect women, but to a great extent, men as well. It's not surprising then that certain sexual acts are viewed as acceptable whereas others are 'kinky' or worse yet 'dirty' or taboo. Rigorous enforcement of religious belief systems too implies that sex is blasé or sinful, and we should strive to overcome it. All this conditioning results in women who believe that it is sinful, wrong and bad for them to seek out and enjoy sex. Not just that, but they believe that they deserve negative consequences and even punishment for daring to do so.

c) Mother-Daughter Bonds and Guilt About Breaking Them

This factor is not so well-known. For most young girls, their mothers are the ones they observe and imitate. As such, they are supremely uncomfortable with doing something that is different from what their role models do. This becomes even more apparent when it comes to a subject such as sex. If a mother is sexually repressed, her daughter will generally find it very difficult to go beyond her mother's boundaries when it comes to sexual fulfillment. The fear and guilt get transferred to other women with the result that most women do not want to stand out as sexually mature individuals.

d) Fear of Arousing Repressed Sadness

When women are in a sexual situation that is also emotionally intimate, they can experience sadness related to some childhood emotional pain. This becomes more acute for women who have experienced rejection or mistreatment early on in life. Such negative experiences are an absolute contrast to the feeling of being not only loved but also pleasured and fulfilled sexually. As such, women can experience very painful emotional responses while making love. If they try to hold these feelings back, they become cut off and detached from the sexual experience.

e) Fear of vulnerability

While women are as capable of initiating and enjoying casual sexual encounters, when they start becoming more involved in a relationship they find that the love and positive acknowledgement can disturb their equilibrium psychologically speaking. These emotions can actually breach their defenses and leave them feeling acutely vulnerable. It brings to the fore that their happiness is dependent upon someone else. As such, they realize that they are wide open to emotional hurt and pain. If they have been hurt before, both men and women are very leery of courting such pain again by making themselves vulnerable. Thus, they hold themselves back during the sexual act and, in women, that can lead to an inability to climax.

f) Abuse and Trauma

It has been estimated that one in every four women has been through inappropriate sexual contact either with strangers or with a relative or family members before she turned 18. As such, they can find themselves sub-consciously linking any sexual experience to their abuser, especially when the abuser is a relative, friend or family member – someone they thought they could trust. In such cases, sex becomes linked to feelings of guilt, revulsion and pain both physical and emotional and therefore, becomes unacceptable to a woman's mind. Unfortunately, such memories can be triggered through a position, things said during sex or even a certain look.

Whew! That's quite a lot, isn't it? The list of factors itself is daunting. Add into this the fact that most women take anywhere between 15 to 40 minutes to climax, and it is a wonder that women ever have an orgasm at all. But that is where you men come in. For the sexual experience to be truly enjoyable, it is essential that both parties enjoy what goes on in the bedroom (or the kitchen, dining room, shower, etc.). As such, we are now going to discuss techniques and positions that will not only help your partner achieve orgasm but also make sure that both of you enjoy the journey thoroughly.

Chapter 3: Types Of Female Orgasms

Yes, gentlemen, you heard right – there are types; and not just one or two, but four types. So for our first lesson in how to make her come, we are going to discuss the different types of orgasms a woman can have and how you can increase her chances to have that orgasm (or those orgasms; whatever, we're not picky).

Clitoral Orgasm

Ah, the clitoris! The confluence of eight thousand nerve endings! For most women, this bundle of nerves is what needs just the right touch to send them tumbling head first into a fantastic orgasm. Having said that, don't head straight for this little bundle. Stimulate other parts of her vagina by caressing and massaging them before you hone in on this little baby.

Techniques – You can make big circles with your fingers that touch upon the clitoral hood, the shaft and the labia. You can do this during foreplay. You can also do this if you're in the spoon position during intercourse. If you are performing oral sex on her, try lying perpendicular to her and thus approach her clitoris indirectly.

Increase her chances – Try using a fingertip vibrator. Encourage her to tell you what setting, speed, pressure and intensity she prefers. Also, try to experiment a bit and take note of her non-verbal cues.

Vaginal Orgasm

It has finally been established. The G-spot exists! This is good news for you lads because 30% of women say that they can come just from having this particular spot stimulated during penetrative sex. Locate, stimulate and enjoy!

Techniques – Of course, the first thing to do is to locate this famous spot. Explore the front wall of her vagina with your finger until you reach a part that feels spongy and rippled in texture. When you touch her there, you will probably see an immediate reaction (a good one). During intercourse, try making sure that you target your thrusting there. You can try lying on your sides facing each other. Intertwine your legs comfortably. Align your genitals and make sure that your penis rubs against the front wall of her vagina. The position ensures deeper thrusts that are more stimulating for the G-spot.

Increase her chances – Her chances of achieving a vaginal orgasm increases the longer the intercourse lasts. Try switching positions often during intercourse. This has a double advantage – it prevents you from coming too soon and helps her experience different and new sensations which can contribute to a vaginal orgasm. Try a warming lubricant for some extra help.

Blended Orgasm

So, as the name suggests, this one mixes the clitoral and the vaginal orgasms. Oh, mama! This one can be a really powerful and explosive finale. In fact, experts say that this is *the most* powerful one. It is estimated that this is twice as intense and strong as either of the other two. She will love you for this one.

Techniques – Girl on top – trust me on this one. There is a reason this one is so popular. It's perfect for this double finish. You can also have her sitting on your lap facing away from you. This way she controls the thrusting while you stimulate the clitoris. If you're doing the missionary, inch your body up so that your hips are aligned. Have her tilt her pelvis upward so that the base of your penis is on the clitoris but the rest of you is inside her. You're not thrusting up and down in this position. Instead, you're grinding against her pelvic bone.

Increase her chances – It's easier for a woman to have a blended orgasm if she becomes very aroused before actual intercourse. Foreplay is king here. You want to do lots of touching, kissing, massaging and licking all over. If you find that the feeling is waning a bit during intercourse, do the heavy petting again.

Multiple Orgasms

The first thing to understand here is what multiple orgasms really are. These are orgasms that happen one right after another. Orgasms that happen at different times during the same session aren't multiple orgasms (although they're still awesome). If your woman can stand being stimulated continuously after the first orgasm (and the second and the third and the fourth and so on), it is possible for her to have multiple orgasms.

Techniques – Start with foreplay. Use your fingers or mouth or a vibrator to get her to her first clitoral climax. Don't stop there, though. Immediately after she comes, you need to continue stimulating her clitoris. For the first 30 seconds do this slowly and then you can resume your normal pace to build her up to a climactic repeat performance. Basically, you're manipulating her level of arousal by easing off a bit when she is more sensitive and then building up the arousal again. From here you can begin intercourse. This can lead to multiple vaginal or even blended orgasms. Remember to use the same technique – slow down, speed up. Keep the stimulation going on and keep the arousal high.

Increase her chances – If she complains about feeling too sensitive, you can use a buffer. Stroke her over a buffer such as a pair of soft silk panties or a silk camisole. You can shift to her breasts and nipples for some time. These areas are quite sensitive, and you can push her to another orgasm simply by stimulating these areas.

Well, there you have it – four basic types of orgasms that women can have and how you can ensure that they have them. Don't think that you are required to master one or the other. The idea here is to explore and find what works for both you and her (especially her!). I hope you find this instructive (and fun – don't forget the fun!).

Chapter 4: Make Her Come

Finally, the chapter you've all been waiting for. In this one, we're going to look at how you can utilize each and every minute of your sexy time with her to ensure she is well taken care of and truly satisfied. Research at the Kinsey Institute shows that on average women take about ten to twenty minutes to climax. We're going to discuss some techniques that'll help you make sure she's still experiencing the aftermath of explosive orgasms well after your 15-minute quickie is over. Not only will it make you a sex god, but research also shows that a woman who has more orgasms will demand more sexy times with you (naturally!).

There is no rule that says you can't cheat a bit – and anyway, it isn't cheating if you don't touch. Subconscious foreplay is fair play. Meet up with her on a day when she has a yoga class, or take her out to a funny movie or a standup comedy show. Have some drinks at your place (or her place – whatever you've decided). Research shows that women are more aroused after they drink a glass or two of red wine. Set the mood and let's begin.

Kiss, Kiss, Kiss

Spend at least three minutes on kissing her thoroughly. Did you know that kissing actually reduces levels of cortisol, also known as the stress hormone, in your body? The more you kiss, the less stressed you are and the easier and faster it is for both of you to get turned on. Tilting your head to the right makes you seem more caring and makes her feel a connection with you. This, in turn, increases oxytocin in her system which encourages her to trust you and thus eventually come faster. Don't spend your time thinking about all this, though. Just enjoy the kiss!

There's More to Kissing than Just the Mouth

In a study of about fifty thousand women, 96 percent said that a kiss on the neck was the perfect way to warm up. Too much isn't good, though – the neck can become desensitized if you only focus there. Kiss her mouth and occasionally slide down to her neck.

At this point, you need to become coordinated. Every time you move down to kiss her neck, remove an item of clothing (hers definitely, yours maybe). Not only does this save you some time, but it also helps you deal with any body-confidence issues that she might have. Remember what we said earlier about how a woman can let her body issues interfere with her ability to enjoy her time with you? Well, this is the perfect way for you to ensure that you show *and* tell her that you love her body. As you remove her clothing, be sure to run your fingertips all over her body, around every curve and dimple she has to subconsciously reassure her mind you appreciate every inch of her body. Add in compliments as you remove each item of clothing. She will feel less self-conscious with each expression of your admiration and approval. Soon, you'll have the tigress you want in your bed (or her bed; again, not picky).

Tease Her Before You Please Her

Building the anticipation is super important. You've probably got most of her clothes off by now. Don't remove her underwear just yet. Yes, I know – it's tempting to head straight in. But patience brings rewards. Tease her by acting as though you have all the time in the world (which you do; this isn't a 100-meter dash). Build up the anticipation both in her and in yourself. Then remove her underwear. It's probably a good idea to use some scented lube at this point as it will excite her and sensitize her at the same time. Remember what we discussed earlier about clitoral orgasms. This is when you want to move your fingers in slow circles around and just inside her vagina.

Oral is Vital

Yes, boys, it is! Research shows that 80 percent of women say that it is the most reliable way for them to achieve the big O. Here's something called the Kivin Method that should get her there in a jiffy. Use one hand to pull up her clitoral hood. Lick the base of the hood, just above the clitoris, from side to side. In the meantime, put one finger of the other hand on the area just below her vaginal opening. You'll know that your finger is in the right place when you feel her pre-orgasmic contractions.

Entrance Exam

While foreplay is a crucial factor in her orgasm, it isn't the only one. Now that you have stimulated her to her first orgasm, intercourse is the next step since the length of the intercourse can determine the consistency of her orgasms. A study in the Journal of Sexual Medicine states that on an average she will climax about seven minutes after penetration. Therefore, now is the time to get started.

Worried about positions? Recall what we discussed about coital alignment technique. To recap, start in the missionary position. Then align your groins in such a way that the base of your penis rests on her clitoris. You want to grind against her pelvic bone, so try a backward and forward movement rather than a thrusting one. This not only massages her clitoris but also gives pulsating and slow sensations that are controlled by you.

You can also try the technique we discussed for the blended orgasm in the previous chapter by spooning her and using your hand or a toy to stimulate her clitoris while thrusting against her G-spot from behind.

Keep it Up

Oh yeah, don't change anything at this point. She should be going wild by now. You don't need anything new to get to the finishing point. You're doing it so just keep on doing it. Keep the speed and pressure the same and once the screaming, clawing climax is over, catch your breath because she's going to want more very soon.

Chapter 5: Positions That Will Work For Her Every Time

So now that we've covered the sex guide to make sure that her experiences with you leave her wanting more (and more and...), we can mix things up a bit. The same old, same old can get exactly that – old. You need to change things up from time to time, not just for her but for you too. At this point, I have to tell you a girl secret (that may not be a secret at all). Most women fake their orgasms – a lot. We know you want to please us, and we don't want to disappoint you. So we fake our orgasm or we just let you assume that we had one. But you don't have to settle for fake when you can blow her mind by giving her the real thing. Here are some positions you can try that will make her explode (in a good way) every time.

1. **Missionary**

    Yes, that's right gentleman. The good old missionary is the one that works best for us. We get the most pleasure out of this old-fashioned position. It's close, it's intimate, it makes us feel cared for because your weight is on us and you surround us. You can make it even better for us by entering at the perfect angle. Don't come straight in. Instead, try a more diagonal approach. It achieves friction for the clitoris which is the best way to make a woman achieve orgasm.

2. **Reverse Cowgirl**

In this position, you are either in a sitting position or lying down. She straddles you backwards, meaning, she faces your feet instead of your head. This position allows you easy access to her clitoris and still gives her control over the thrusts. Not only will this get her a clitoral orgasm, but you can also even give her a blended one.

3. Doggy Style

This position is not just great for the man; it is also brilliant for the woman. It gives her a good amount of control. She can determine what angle is best for her and adjust her range of motion accordingly. You can stimulate her G-spot and her clitoris. Use your hand or a toy such as a small bullet vibrator. Don't just leave it up to the toy, though. Your hand is very important because remember, it's all about touch.

4. Girl on Top

This position is again a favorite because it allows her control of her own orgasm. This is basically the reverse of reverse cowgirl, so she's straddling you and facing your head. Encourage her to move in a backwards and forward motion instead of an up and down one – more stimulation for her clitoris. Don't just lie there, though. Join in by moving her hips. It gives more of an in sync feeling and makes for better communication – you know what she wants, and she knows what you want. Both of you work towards it together.

5. Spooning

In case she doesn't enjoy deep penetration (it can happen), try spooning. The efficacy of this technique can be seen in the fact that I've already mentioned it twice, and I'm talking about it again. It's fairly relaxed, so if you're into a lazy weekend morning play session, this position is perfect. The stimulation happens in the front wall of the vagina – yes that's right, the G-spot. At the same time, you can go for a blended orgasm by stimulating her clitoris.

6. Crisscross

This one is another great one if you want to focus on clitoral stimulation. Both of you need to lie down. You should be on your side, while she is on her back. Her legs are draped over your middle, kind of like a giant X. Either one of you can reach down and stimulate her clitoris since you're not squeezed against each other.

7. The Pillow Technique

It has been found by various sex experts and researchers that a woman finds sex more pleasurable when a pillow or a blanket is added into the mix because it makes for a new and different angle of entry. You can use the pillow in the missionary position by putting it under her bottom to raise her pelvis. This can help you stimulate her G-spot upon penetration. Not every angle will be comfortable for her so find out what works for her and use that.

8. Coital Alignment Technique

You knew I was going to bring this baby back! Just like the spooning, this is a great position to ensure mutual enjoyment and fulfillment. Some have even called it the 'greatest sexual position in the world'. It was created by psychotherapist Edward Eichel and involves you lying in missionary not resting your weight on your arms. You need to move so that the base of your penis is in direct contact with her clitoris. Remember to lock her legs around your thighs. Use a rocking rather than a thrusting motion. This position works out great not just because of the clitoral stimulation but also because it is physically the closest position.

9. Ankles Up

Moving her legs around can help because sometimes being on top of her or flat on her will not give you the penetration both of you need. In this position, you put her ankles up on your shoulders. This allows for a much deeper penetration and ensures you hit her G-spot with every thrust. You can also do this by bending her knees or putting her feet flat on your chest.

10. Kneeling

This is another woman on top position. You sit in an armchair or on the bed, and she kneels on the chair or bed, straddling you. She controls not just the penetration but also when both of you will climax by deciding the speed, grind and thrust to suit her own (and your) pace. Even if she isn't someone who wants to be in control, she can still enjoy the position if you take charge and move her around to suit you.

11. Edge of the Bed

This one is similar to the ankles up position in that it encourages deeper penetration. In the edge of the bed position, she lies on her back, and her hips are at the edge of the bed. You enter from under her legs. She can let them drop off the edge or rest them on your torso. Before you try this position, keep in mind the height of the bed and whether your groin will be in line with hers or not. You might need to bend or lower yourself a bit in order to penetrate her completely. The feel is sexy though because it suggests an urgency and impatience – as though you couldn't wait to get on to the bed properly. Not only that, she gets to view all the action, which, trust me, is hot!

12. Cowgirl with a Twist

Alright, so this is cowgirl but a bit more than just that. She assumes the cowgirl position, straddling you and facing your head. Then you raise your knees so as to support her bottom. She can, then, push off your chest and slide up and down against your thighs. Be warned, though – the lady controls when you climax so she can delay it if she wants. You want her to get there though so this shouldn't be a problem. To add spice, meet each of her thrusts by grabbing on to her thighs or hips.

13. The Bridge

So, this one starts out innocently enough with the missionary position. Then you need to sit up and ensure that your weight is supported on your ankles. Your knees need to be spread wide for balance. She should lie on her back with her feet flat on the bed. Then, she should arch her hips up so that she's in a low bridge position. This way you get the perfect angle for penetration and the maximum amount of penetration. If she finds the position uncomfortable, you can put some pillows under her back to prop it up.

14. Belly Down

Alright, this is a slightly new one compared to what we've discussed before and the sensations generated are new too. She goes on the bottom, face-down. You are on top either lying on top of her or utilizing a sort of a semi-push up position. Then you enter her. She needs to keep her legs straight and her hips slightly raised to facilitate the penetration. This works out great for both of you. Your penis is straight in line with her G-spot so you hit it on every thrust. She is super snug, so you get a great tight fit. Use a water based lube to ensure that everything glides into position as smoothly as possible. You can raise her hips by propping pillows under her pelvic region or vagina, especially if you're having a problem with alignment due to different heights.

15. Standing Against a Wall

This one is a classic quickie position. It is also one of oldest positions for a quickie. For it to work best, she needs to be the one against the wall. She needs to lean her pelvis forward, and her shoulders and back should be braced against the wall for support. Then she should wrap her leg around your waist. This controls your penetration and speed. The two requirements for this position to work out well are: the two partners should be of similar height, and she should have strong leg muscles. If there is a significant height difference, you may find it challenging to penetrate her.

16. Bent at the Waist

This one involves you standing behind her, while bends at the waist, as the name suggests and you enter her from behind. This position makes her vaginal walls tighter and therefore increases the friction. It doesn't hurt that this is an easy angle for penetration. Don't just expect her to bend without support, though – that could quickly become uncomfortable for her. Instead, ensure that there is something in front for her to hold on to such as a table, the back of a chair or a couch or even a sink. If she has that support, it leaves your hands free – you can use one hand to hold on to her and the other to reach around and rub her clitoris.

17. Missionary with a Twist

This one involves you getting into the missionary position and then, as the name says, turning onto your side – both of you. You need to use your arms to support each other and intertwine your legs so that you get a better fit and more leverage. You stay connected to each other the entire time. You move very slowly and roll to the side while still having intercourse. Of course, the clitoral stimulation doesn't let up which obviously is very important for her to reach the big O.

18. Cross-Legged

A common misconception about this position is that you need to be very flexible to be able to pull it off. While sitting in a cross-legged like a pretzel position is great, it's not necessary. All you really need is to sit cross legged so that your erection points upwards. She will sit facing you in your lap and wrap her legs around your waist or your hips. This works for both of you because you get maximum penetration while she controls the thrusts by riding or rocking. She can hold on to your shoulders for support.

19. The Spider

In this position, both of you need to be sitting on the bed, facing each other. Lean back on your hands for support. Your legs should be pointed towards one another. She needs to walk her feet over your body and to the sides of your hips and place her feet flat on the bed. This position allows you to penetrate her perfectly. Don't thrust into her; rock back and forth. The best part is that you can look at each other and at the action going on and she gets to control the motion, speed and angle to get to her climax.

20. The Pretzel

Again you don't have to be a flexible practitioner of the most difficult yoga that you can find to do this. This one is actually a mix of Doggy Style and face to face. She needs to lie down on her left side. Then you straddle her left leg, and she wraps her right leg around your waist.

Feel free to determine what works best for both of you in this one.

So, I've listed twenty positions that guarantee pleasure not just for you but for her every time. Once you are comfortable with these positions, go ahead and experiment to see what works out best for both of you. Talk to each other about what worked and what didn't. If you find a position particularly difficult, try practicing with each other while fully clothed. Spontaneity is all well and good, but sometimes practice is better – after all, it does make perfect.

Chapter 6: Additional Tips To Help Both Of You Out

We've discussed techniques, positions and procedures. We've tried to understand the history of the female orgasm, what influences it and how to achieve it. While techniques and positions are great, remember that a woman orgasms as much from her mind as she does from her body. To help her get there, you need to ensure that her brain enjoys the experience as much as her body does. Here are some additional tips to help you get brain and body in sync and take her to the ultimate explosion.

Stop Worrying About Time

Your worry is about how long you may last. For her, the worry is about whether she's taking too long. As I've mentioned earlier, women do take longer to achieve an orgasm than do men. Having said that, it is very possible that she feels self-conscious about how long she's taking to get there and therefore ends up faking an orgasm rather than making it to the finish line.

To help her out with this one, take the pressure off her and yourself. Tell her that she and you have the whole night to get where both of you need to go. She needs to relax to be able to have an orgasm at all. So, let her do that and focus on the journey. Show her that not only are you in it for the long haul and that you like (as in really like) her sexual responses. The better she feels about this, the more likely she is to achieve climax.

Use Your Talent

Whatever it may be, it'll turn her on. Croon 'Careless Whisper' or show her your etchings (before you show her your 'etchings'). Studies at the Kinsey Institute show that talent is actually a greater turn on for women than chiseled abs or film-star good looks. If humor is your forte, use it. Connect with her on this level and she'll feel more comfortable with you and more attracted to you.

Tell Her What You Like About Her Body

Again, as I've mentioned earlier, body issues can become a great big roadblock on the way to orgasmic bliss for her. To reassure her and remove this roadblock, tell her what you like about her body. You don't have to make stuff up – after all, you do like her naked, right? Just tell her.

Be Gentle Up Top

More than the areola and the nipples, the top, bottom and sides of her breasts are sensitive. Gently brush your fingers, hands and lips on these areas. Pay close attention to her responses. Slowly build up to the nipples. Once the arousal builds, her nipples are ready for your attention and so is she.

Learn What Strokes Play Her Just Right

Remember, we women like a slow buildup. Hard and fast doesn't always work out so well for us. Here's a way you can build up the stimulation. Lying next to her, place the heel of one hand just above her clitoris. Next, you need to run your middle finger and your ring finger along her outer lips. Start with a feather touch and then build the pressure up. Use your palm to cup the area around her clitoris so that the sensation builds up. Don't try to touch the clitoris directly in the beginning. It's a sensitive bundle, and most women won't be ready for the sensation of direct stimulation. As her arousal builds up, you can brace your hand on her pubic mound or her mons and use the tips of your fingers to tease her clitoris while moving your hand.

Try a Different Angle

Tried and tested is fine for a while but make sure that you keep things fresh and interesting. Try different positions and different angles of penetration to see what works for her and you. Remember to use positions and angles that hit her G-spot every time. You can even use your fingers to massage the area. If a particular position or angle doesn't work for her, don't sweat it; just move on.

Multitasking is Hot

To ensure maximum pleasure for her, try out moves that bring you in contact with several of her sensitive zones at the same time. For example, you can have her lie on her back. She should stretch out her legs. Get on top and curl your arms around her shoulders. Use your elbows to support yourself and bring your chest level with her chin. This is another way you can achieve the oft-mentioned and very successful coital alignment technique.

Watch Out for Signs of Her Orgasm

When you start oral sex, don't go hell for leather right from the outset. Remember, gentle and slow build up is the key here. Don't even start with her vagina. Try her hips and then move to her thighs and then her inner thighs. Different women are sensitive in different parts so figure that out. Then move to her outer and inner lips and kiss them. Finally, move inside using broad and firm strokes of your tongue.

Throughout all of this, watch and listen to determine what she likes and what she loves. Listen to her moans and cries. See how her hips move. You can tell when she's close to orgasm by the changing color of her labia, which happens because of increased blood flow. You can also put your hand on her stomach to check for the contractions that happen immediately before her orgasm.

Follow Her Lead

This is where things are different for men and women. When you start on the road to your climax, nothing and I mean nothing will derail you (short of the possibility of Lorena Bobbitt appearing in your bedroom). Unfortunately, the same is not true for your lady. While changing positions midway to the big O might not affect your arousal, it could ring the death knell for hers. Try new things; just not when she's about to explode. The whole thing will end up a complete anti-climax for her (pun definitely intended).

Let the Lady Go First

Be a gentleman here and let her hit her orgasm first. While it's great that you want both of you to come together, let's face it, that doesn't always work out. Chances are you'll hit the goal first, and she'll be left far behind in your wake. Too much rubbing of the clitoris can even desensitize it, killing any chance of her achieving an orgasm. So, ensure she has come at least once before intercourse.

An added bonus here is that once she's come for the first time, her orgasm threshold will drop. This means that it's easier for you to bring her to climax a second or a third time.

Chapter 7: Myths About Female Orgasms

Unfortunately, despite a much more open attitude towards female sexuality and orgasms than society has had in the past, there are plenty of myths still doing the rounds. A lot of information out there is bad or compared to male orgasms which actually happen very differently. In this chapter, I'll undertake the busting of some of these myths and hope that you, my gentlemen readers, are not led astray by them.

1. **Orgasm is the End Goal of Sex**

    No, no and a thousand times no. My vehemence about this point is because it puts too much pressure on both the partners to achieve and help each other achieve orgasm. An activity that is really about pleasure and intimacy becomes a race to the finish. Instead, take time out to explore each other (ladies, I'm looking at you too) and learn what works for both of you. Try out something new or just a variation of something tried and tested. Take pleasure in being with each other, even if this is something you've done a gazillion times before.

2. **Multiple Orgasms Are Easy for All Women**

    Nope, not true. Yes, we do have the capacity for multiple orgasms (lucky us). But most women actually don't have them, regardless of what the movies say. Even the women who do have them don't achieve them easily and don't have them every time. Typically, women who have multiple orgasms have trained themselves, or their partners, to hit their pleasure spots just right every time. This is not something that will just happen, so give her and yourself some time to learn what works for both of you.

3. All Women like Romantic Movie Sex

Umm, not always. While gentle and tender is nice, we like getting it hard and rough too (find out before you try it though). Sometimes, the mood is just not right for romance, but it is right for hard, pure sex. We do enjoy that just as much as men do, you know.

4. Safer Sex Isn't Sexier Sex

Ok, this one is just plain crazy. We think ourselves into orgasms, remember? Do you really think a woman will be able to come if she's worrying about a potential baby or a sexually transmitted infection or disease? Besides, you using protection shows us you care about our safety and well-being, and that is sexy.

5. Skilled Partner Means No Sex Toys

Actually, a partner is skilled if he knows how to bring a woman to a climax. As such, using sex toys to maximize her pleasure actually shows off his skill. His mad skills and toys both? Ooh la la!

6. All Women Can Orgasm Easily

All I'm going to say about this one is that if this statement were true, this e-book wouldn't be necessary.

7. **Penetration is Needed For a Woman to Orgasm**

   As the techniques discussed in this book shows, this one is simply not true. Clitoral stimulation is what leads to female orgasm most of the time, and penetration is not needed to stimulate a woman's clitoris. Since there are different types other than a penetration orgasm, we'll just leave it at that.

8. **You will go blind or hair will grow on your palms**

This was created in order to shame people so that they would not please themselves because it made them think that they were going to end up with a physical deformity. However, as we can tell from thousands of years of people pleasing themselves, this is a complete lie!

9. **If you orgasm while masturbating, you cannot orgasm while having actual sex.**

As long as you do not allow for your masturbation schedule to get in the way of having orgasms with your partner, then you have nothing to worry about! In fact, when you are having sex with your partner and trying to reach that glorious end, you can use toys or masturbation during sex in order to climax if you are having trouble.

10. **You are in a relationship, you do not need to be masturbating.**

Well, masturbating is actually been found to help women show their partner's what it is that they like for when their partners go to touch them. And as we just mentioned, touching yourself during sex can actually assist in bringing on your orgasm. And last but not least, do people think that you are going to just sit around and wait for sex if your partner is out of town? I wouldn't! Why not spice things up and touch yourself while you are on the phone with your partner? It will definitely help with the orgasm when your partner does return because they know exactly what they have been missing!

Chapter 8: Solo Play

Sometimes when push comes to shove you have to take things into your own hands. Solo paly is going to be the best way for you to be able to tell your partner how you like it and how to reach your orgasm!

When you are playing alone, you can use your hands or toys whichever way you find that you are going to be able to find that you are reaching your final destination. Sometimes, it also helps to make up fantasies when you are doing solo play because it is going to give you something to focus on, such as that hot actor's hands all over your body in ways that no one else has ever touched you before!

Masturbation tips

1. Get into the mood! Nothing is worse than when you are trying to get off and you find that you are not in the mood. So, making sure that you are in the proper mood is going to be the number one thing. However, only you are going to know if you are in the mood for your play time or not.

Some people do not take much to get into the mood, all they need to do is pull out the toys or lay in bed. Other people have to drag it out and make it elaborate so that they feel special before they are able to start.

2. Privacy. Nothing is more embarrassing than someone walking in on what you are doing! It is the fastest way for a mood to be killed. So, no matter

where you are, make sure that you can lock the door so that no one is coming in on you. If you do not feel comfortable masturbating when there are other people in the house, then you should wait till there is no one there and you are going to have a little bit of time to yourself in order to allow yourself time to be vocal.

It is also a good idea to keep your phone off, on silent, or even in the other room so that it is not breaking your concentration.

3. Focus on your clitoris. As you are working on your solo play, you are going to come to realize that having a clitoral orgasm is going to be a lot easier to achieve than a vaginal orgasm. This is especially going to help when you are first learning how to masturbate.

The first thing that you need to know is that your clitoris is the small bundle of nerves that gets bigger the more aroused that you are. It can be located above your vagina and under a small fold of skin that will be extremely sensitive after you have found your climax.

When you are wanting to stimulate your clit, you are going to rub it with your fingers. For some women, this is the best way to get your orgasm. But, others find that it is going to give them more stimulation by using indirect stimulation so they do not touch it directly, they rub around it to make it more sensitive. You may want to massage it slowly before you begin to get rough with it so that you are able to build your climax up and so that you are getting your body use to a new source of stimulation.

4. Gspots are another great way to have an orgasm. Sadly, many people do not know where their gspot is because it is only going to be found when it is engorged which is going to happen when you are aroused.

The gspot is going to be located inside of your vagina on the front wall. It is going to be slightly rough to the touch but it is going to be similar to running your tongue across the top of your mouth.

Gspot stimulation comes in many different forms such as inserting your fingers into your vagina and curling them into a come-hither motion thus allowing your fingers to press against it. From there, you are going to be able to masturbate how you find comfortable. Other ways are to use toys but the toys are going to be your own decision because what works for you may not work for your best friend.

5. Lube. It may seem a little out there to use lube when you are masturbating but lube is not just to use with another person. there are different types of lubes that are going to amp up that pleasurable feeling. You are going to have to experiment to find out which lube is right for you.

6. Toys toys everywhere! If all else fails, one of the best ways to make your orgasm more intense is to use toys. There are many different toys that are on the

market and the one that works best for you is the one that you are going to find that you cannot live without.

For many, a vibrator is all that they need because they are able to adjust the speed and place the pulsing toy next to their clit or in their vagina and find that perfect spot that sends them towards a screaming oh. However, you have to be careful with some vibrators because they tend to get stuck at a high speed and then become too strong.

Dildos are another option and are great for whenever your partner is not there. Some dildos even going to double as a vibrator and can reach places that fingers never will be able to.

Last but not least, you can use a butt plug. There are some women in the world that have said having something in their behind make their orgasm more intense. This is not going to be true for every woman, but it is going to be true for some.

7. Porn is not just for guys. For some porn gives the proper images and noises that make it to where you are able to find your orgasm. Sometimes you do not have to watch it, just the noises help. But, there are all variations of porn out there and you have to find what works best for you.

8. Erotic stories are going to allow you to create your own images. But they are not going to be for everyone. If you do not find anything else that works, this is one thing to try.

9. Keep learning!! There is always more that you can learn about your body and masturbation. Pick up a book, search online and you will find what you are looking for that works for you.

Techniques to use when you are masturbating

1. Up and down: this one is pretty easy and it is going to focus mainly on your clit. Take however many fingers you want to use and rub up and down beside your clit. If you are wanting more simulation, you can rub your clit directly.

2. Long slow stroke: still using your fingers, you are going to go from the middle of your clit to the bottom of your vagina. You are going to find which areas of your vagina make you jerk and which ones your body does not like. do not ignore your body and do things that your body does not like or you are not going to reach your orgasm.

3. Side to side: just like when you were going up and down, on your clit. But this time you are going to go side to side. When you are using this technique you can also include

    a. Switching directions

    b. Using indirect contact

    c. Different speeds

    d. The number of fingers that you use

- e. The pressure you are using
- f. Lube

4. Fun with four fingers: you are going to use four fingers to go over your clit in order to stimulate your climax. You are going to hold your four fingers togheer and rub them around your clit and vagina. You can do circles or you can go side to side depending on what you prefer. This is also going to stimulate your uspot.

5. Uspot: your uspot is going to be slightly lower than your clit and is above the urethral opening. When you are wanting to stimulate it, you will stroke it with just the tip of your finger. The softer that you rub it along with rubbing your clit, the more stimulation you are going to experience.

6. Shower head love: do not be afraid to admit it, using the shower head or the faucet is a great way to get off. If you have yet to do it, then you are going to want to get to it because it is one of the best methods to use for masturbation!

You are not going to have to use your fingers if you do not want to and you are going to be able to get the entirety of your vagina so that you can find the perfect spot. With the shower head, you can change the pressure of the water, how far away it is from your vagina, or the temperature of the water to find your orgasm.

7. Under the hood: you may or may not have noticed that you have a clitoris that is super sensitive. Not all

women have this, but when it is sensitive, it can sometimes be pleasurable to touch so you have to find other ways to masturbate.

One of the methods that you can use is to use the hood of your clitoris as a butter so that you are not touching your clitoris directly.

8. Hood life: there are other women whose clit is not sensitive at all and they have to move the hood of their clitoris. Women like this usually have to rub and grind in order to get their clitoris stimulated. Instead, you can always move the hood and get straight to your clitoris without any harm.

9. Orgasmic mediation: for this technique, you are going to lay on your back and spready our legs so that they are not harming you, but you can easily get to your vagina. You are then going to stroke your clitoris and various other parts of your vagina.

You can also do this with a partner and have your partner sit to your right with his left leg over your stomach holding you down slightly with his other leg under your right leg.

10. The squeeze: when using the squeeze, you are going to be focusing on your clitoris. The first thing that you are going to do is place your thumb and index finger on either side of your clit. From there you are going to squeeze starting with a gentle pressure and upping the pressure until you are able to stimulate your clit into an orgasm.

11. Lovely Labia: as you rub on your labia it is a good source of foreplay and if done right, you will achieve an orgasm. Some ways you can add to rubbing your labia are:

    a. Running different materials over it

    b. Run your fingers up and down it

    c. Use lube for a silky feeling.

    d. Squeeze your fingers together.

12. Use a pillow: some women like to hump or grind in order to get their orgasm. Things like toys, blankets, and pillows are good for this technique so you can stimulate your clitoris and labia at the same time.

    a. Use your partner's thigh

    b. Lie on your side with a pillow between your legs. Squeezing your legs together, and pull the pillow between your legs so it is pressing against all your gooey parts before beginning to grind

    c. Put a towel over your pillow and grind on that so that you get a different feeling. Not only are you keeping your pillow dry, but you can try other things like toys or electric toothbrushes.

    d. A small pillow can be folded in half to achieve the same effect if you do not have a long pillow.

13. Pearl necklace: when doing pearl necklace, you will take beads of some sort between your legs. You will lay on your back and place the beads so that they are across your entire vagina. You will pull the beads up and down slowly to stimulate yourself. Some lube on the beads makes it to where you are not having such a rough surface.

You can also use a towel or silk scarf for this method. However, do not use anything too expensive just in the event it breaks.

14. Vibrators are great if you cannot get any of these methods to work. There are so many kinds of vibrators out there that you are going to have to experiment and find the one that works best for you. There are vibrators that are no bigger than the tip of your finger and then there are ones that you have to plug into the wall. But in the end, they are all going to give you the explosion that you want.

If you are too scared to go to a sex toy store that is in your area, you are able to order them offline. However, when you order offline you are not going to be able to tell if that is the proper one for you. Getting a feel for the vibrator is part of what tells you if it is the one for you or not.

Ultimately, there are several different ways that you are going to be able to get off when you are masturbating, it is up to you to find the way that works best. If you want to masturbate while your partner watches, then that is completely your choice because this is about you! Go on and get your orgasm because you deserve it!

Chapter 9: Getting the Best Orgasm of Your Life

Getting off can sometimes be hard because of things that get in the way such as muscle cramps! However, if you are wanting to experience that mystical gem that is known as the multiple orgasms, or even just get your first orgasm, there are a few things that you are going to want to know so that you can get the best orgasm of your life.

- Coregasms: there is always more than one way to get to your orgasm and the path that you choose is going to be the one that is best for you. However, one thing that most people do not understand is that you can reach your orgasm by exercising! Research has proven that some women have an orgasm by having pelvic muscle contractions and tightening up their legs and abdominal muscles as they are working out. Having an orgasm and losing weight? Sign me up!

- Birthgasms: it does not happen to many, but there have been some women that find an orgasm when they are in the middle of labor. Like we just mentioned, it is the tightening of those abdominal muscles and the pelvic contractions that lead you to it. But, think about who you have in the birthing room just in case this happens to you. There is nothing more embarrassing than getting off in front of your mother in law.

- Thoughts: it has been found that the correct amount of visualization, giving yourself permission, and counting will allow you to have an orgasm in their own head. It is a great way to practice your orgasms so that you can achieve them when you are in bed.

- Volume: adding in things like high pitched noises or low pitch can also affect your orgasm. The high-pitched noises are going to increase the sexual energy that is coursing through your head, chest, and throat. Obviously, the pitches are going to impact your lower half and bring you to that magical moment.

- Pillow talk: meeting your end releases oxytocin in your brain which makes your emotions heightened. Depending on whole you just got done doing the nasty with depends on if you want to have pillow talk. If it is just a random hook up, stick to the spooning so you are not saying something you regret later on.

Every woman is not the same! So, what works for one will not work for another all the time. Not to mention your nationality is going to play a part in how many times you do the nasty.

Conclusion

So here we are at the end of the journey. I hope that you gentlemen have learned more about women and their orgasms and feel more confident about being able to please your partners. You should now be aware of how the female orgasm has been perceived throughout history. You also know the factors that affect the ability of a woman to achieve an orgasm during sexual intercourse.

I hope you now understand the different types of orgasms women can have and how you can ensure that they receive them. If you go through the fifteen-minute quickie guide, it can actually act as a blueprint for pretty much all of your sexual encounters, no matter how much time you intend to take over them. All that varies is how much time you would spend on each of the steps I've outlined. Remember to switch things up, because variety is the spice of life! It'll keep your sex life happy and interesting long after your first encounter with your partner. The different positions I've outlined in Chapter 5 should help both of you enjoy a great time in bed and out of it. Just keep in mind that it is all about the journey and not the destination. Take pleasure in each other and in giving each other pleasure and the orgasms will take care of themselves.

I've also added a few tips that I think you will find useful, not only in terms of physical stimulation but also in terms of mental reassurance and comfort. Women's orgasms are as much a product of their minds as of their bodies. Remember to keep the mind as relaxed as possible so that the body can enjoy the sexual act. Listen to the cues your partner gives you, both verbal and physical and use those to determine what works for her and what doesn't.

I hope that you enjoyed this book and took away something useful from it. If you would be willing to leave a review about this book, I would be very grateful. Thank you very much for purchasing and reading my book. I wish you many healthy, safe and happy sexual encounters.